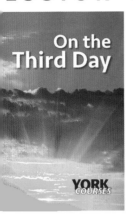

On the Third Day

YORK COURSES

AVE I GOT EWS FOR YOU!

we ggest you read the main xt first, and then come ack to the margin boxes. rhaps mark a couple of e quotations you might e to discuss.

> Jesus loves me this I now, for the Bible tells ne so.
>
> *Karl Barth, Protestant theologian*

believe in the esurrection because have seen it and xperienced it in my own fe. It is the death of the ld self and the rebirth f the new self which is t the very heart of the hristian drama.

Giles Fraser, priest and journalist

C000181230

Mr Wrigley was a no-nonsense sidesman in our chur the hymn books with smile. He didn't say n coffee. But once a yea Day he would walk fr all the way to the vica doorway and say to t the vicar would reply, 'He is risen indeed, Mr Wrigley.' Mr Wrigley would nod, satisfied with the answer, and then walk all the way to the back of the church for the rest of the year.

I used to love that exchange. Here was this undemonstrative Christian man bearing witness to the core belief that kept him going in life. He could continue giving out hymn books, and doing his job, and loving his wife, and paying his taxes, because Christ was risen and so everything else would be all right.

It's the faith that has motivated countless millions of people on every continent for two thousand years. It's the faith that has given a foundation to whole nations. It's the faith that continues to propel the Church into a world of uncertainty and need. It's the faith that moved me from a 'don't know' to a joyful 'yes!'

But I have a sneaking suspicion that many Christians would prefer not to be asked to give their reasons for believing in the resurrection. After all, it can be taken as read that dead people don't rise from a grave. How can intelligent people think otherwise? What kind of fairy story is this?

Of course, no-one saw the resurrection actually happen, and in any case the resurrection is more a mystery to enter into than a fact to put on a dissecting table. Nevertheless, the important thing about pursuing truth is that we have to enter the chase with an open mind and not decide *a priori* that something couldn't be the case. You have to look at the data.

There are at least five pieces of evidence to look at. The first is:

1. The empty tomb. All the gospels report this as an incontrovertible fact. The question is: 'why is it empty?' Well, who else might have moved the body? If it were the disciples wanting to keep this precious friend's

The gospels don't explain the resurrection; the resurrection explains the gospels. Belief in the resurrection isn't an appendage to the Christian faith; it is the Christian faith.

John Whale, theologian

'Do you believe in God?'
'Yes.'
'Do you believe in a God who can change the course of events on earth?'
'No, just the ordinary one.'
From an academic survey in Islington in the late 1960s

When Jesus reached the point of no return, he did return.

C F D Moule, New Testament scholar

We aren't immune from suffering or excused from the experience of being human simply because of our faith. And the truth remains: the crucified God, as personified in Jesus, revealed that God is always on the side of suffering wherever it is found and God's endgame is resurrection.

Sarah Bessey, writer

body safe, why would they pursue the falsehood to the point of martyrdom? Why make silly claims? If it were the Jewish leaders or the Romans wanting to avoid a cult of veneration of Jesus, why didn't they produce his body when things started to get out of hand?

The point about veneration is interesting. Such reverence at holy places was commonplace, as it is today at the shrines of, for example, Abraham, St Francis or St Cuthbert. But there is no evidence of Christians gathering at the tomb of Jesus for at least three centuries; they were too busy meeting the risen Lord elsewhere!

We might note, also, that the gospel accounts credit women with being the first witnesses to the empty tomb – precisely those in society least likely to be believed. Not evidence you would make up if you were trying to persuade people to believe. The gospel stories all have the breathless, urgent, dramatic quality of eye-witness accounts. They're devoid of Old Testament references (compared with the accounts of the crucifixion) and so they read as authentic first-hand testimony to a totally new kind of event.

In assessing the truth of the Christian claim about the resurrection, the empty tomb is *necessary* evidence, but it's not *sufficient* in itself. We need more.

2. **The resurrection appearances.** Jesus is reported as having been seen over an extended period of time, by a variety of people, in a variety of places - at the tomb, in the Upper Room, on an evening walk to Emmaus, by the sea-shore in Galilee, on a mountain top, and 'by 500 people at one time' (1 Corinthians 15.6). Was this imagination, hallucination, wish-fulfilment? What do we make of it?

Let's be clear. Jewish believers had no expectation of an individual resurrection; they only envisaged a final resurrection of all the faithful on the last day. So this wasn't wish-fulfilment. Again, they were not simple people; they were used to dreams, but they knew the difference between a dream and a real appearance, something corroborated by the references to Jesus eating with the disciples and inviting Thomas to touch his wounds. So it wasn't hallucination either.

When we celebrate Easter we are really standing in the middle of a second Big Bang, a tumultuous surge of divine energy as fiery and intense as the very beginning of the universe.

*

Jesus is set free, he's not going to die again, nothing prevents him from acting, he is always going to be active and not passive, always at work. And so, to say he is risen is to say he is now free to act eternally, unceasingly, without limit. Death and its effects cannot hold him back.

*

To believe in the resurrection is to believe that Jesus, in the great phrase of John Masefield, is 'alive and at large in the world'.

Rowan Williams, former Archbishop of Canterbury

The great heroes of history seem to be those who have won wars. True success, however, may be those who managed to avoid fighting them.

Daniel Finkelstein, journalist and politician

This is very early testimony. Paul wrote his first letter around 55AD, so no more than 25 years after Jesus died. There would still have been many witnesses alive who could have disproved the claim that: 'Five hundred saw him at one time, most of whom', Paul is careful to point out, 'are still alive'.

I once ate a daffodil in church on Easter Day to make the point that if someone there that morning went home and told their family the vicar ate a daffodil in church, the family would be unlikely to believe it. But if 500 people had said the same thing, they might have to start believing it had actually happened. (No need to say that I was sick immediately afterwards – don't eat the stalk!)

When you put the empty tomb and the sightings of Jesus together you come to a conclusion that seems both necessary *and* sufficient – that this Jesus really had been raised from the dead and was meeting people in real time. But there's more data to bring forward.

3. **The transformation of the disciples.** The gospels and the letters of the New Testament give us remarkable 'before' and 'after' pictures of the disciples. Indeed, it's hard to recognise them as the same people. 'Before' they were broken and demoralised. They'd denied and deserted Jesus; now they were hiding away to avoid the same fate as him. 'After', in the early chapters of Acts, we see them fearlessly and joyfully telling everyone they can about what they've seen and heard. They're arrested, harassed, beaten up, martyred, but they're unstoppable. Something radical has happened. Something big enough to account for their total transformation.

I have a friend who occupied a very senior position in the police force and it was this transformation that convinced him, with all his detective experience, that the resurrection wasn't a myth and that Jesus must have been raised from the dead.

4. **The existence of the Church.** The early Church was soon exploding in size. Within 300 years the might of Rome itself had fallen under the spell of the penniless preacher from Galilee. Now 30% of the

Christianity is based on hope against evidence to the contrary.

Garrison Keillor, broadcaster

I regard the conclusion [that Jesus rose from the dead] as coming in the same sort of category - of historical probability so high as to be virtually certain - as the death of Augustus in AD 14 or the fall of Jerusalem in AD 70.

Tom Wright, New Testament scholar

The whole point, in my radical reading of resurrection, is that the community that is searching for Christ is the living body of Christ … He is here, in our love, already.

Slavoj Žižek, philosopher

In a daring and beautiful reversal, God takes the worst we can do to him, and turns it into the very best he can do for us.

Malcolm Guite, poet and theologian

world's population names the name of Christ and there are 70,000 more believers every day of the year (net growth). Could all of this be based on a lie or a mistake?

5. What they said about Jesus. Within a very few years the people who had known Jesus best, who had walked the paths of Galilee with him, chatted on the way, shared the jokes, the barbeques and the washing-up, these friends of Jesus were speaking of him in terms that applied to God. They were calling him 'Lord', and giving him scores of other exalted names and titles. Paul refers to Jesus as 'Lord' nearly all the time, and that was how Greek-speaking Jews referred to God himself. This was astonishing for fiercely monotheistic Jews. Look at Philippians 2.5-11 to get a flavour of how radical this really was. Again, something huge had caused such a claim, something like a resurrection. Only a risen Christ can justify such extravagance.

Back at the beginning I suggested that the resurrection is more a mystery to enter into than a fact to put on a dissecting table. We're obviously out of our league in terms of understanding this unparalleled event with normal mental apparatus. But that doesn't mean we leave our rational minds in the waiting room. We let evidence and analysis take us as far as they can - and then we go further. The rational may have to give way to the supra-rational, the arena of God's freedom and grace. Yes, we must push the arguments, but ultimately perhaps the instinctive faith of Mr Wrigley has much to commend it.

'Christ is risen, vicar!' 'He is risen indeed, Mr Wrigley.'

We are sometimes asked if it is okay to copy our course materials (booklets, CDs/audio/newspaper articles).
Please don't, as this breaks copyright law.

Evil things often happen because we live in a fallen world of free agents … God is not to blame. I didn't learn how to lament and grieve, how to pray and be in community until I learned that God could be trusted. God is against the evil and suffering in the world.

Sarah Bessey, writer

QUESTIONS FOR GROUPS

BLE READING: John 20.19-28

ome groups will address all the questions. hat's fine. Others prefer to select just a few nd spend longer on each. That's fine, too. lorses for (York) Courses!

Well-loved Bible passages read at Easter include Doubting Thomas (John 20.24-28), Mary Magdalene in the garden (John 20.11-18) and the two disciples on the road to Emmaus (Luke 24.28-35). What is your favourite Easter reading - and why?

Read John 11.25. On p. 1 Bishop John tells us that his new-found belief in the strong evidence for the resurrection of Jesus, moved him from a 'don't know' to a joyful 'yes!' Where do you stand on this spectrum of assurance? Our participants discuss this on track 5 of the audio/transcript.

In a 2017 Com-Res survey for the BBC, 43% of the 2,010 British people asked, said they believed in the Resurrection. Does this figure surprise you? Share your reaction with fellow group members.

Re-read para. 2 of Session 1 and Karl Barth's words in the box on p. 1. Bishop John suggests that faith in the resurrection of Jesus was the 'core belief' that kept Mr Wrigley going. Do you have a 'core belief'? What keeps you going in the ups and downs of life?

Read 1 Peter 3.15. Bishop John says he has a 'sneaking suspicion that many Christians would prefer not to be asked to give their reasons for believing in the Resurrection.' Do you think he's right? Has anyone ever asked you for your reasons? If they did, what would you say?

6. **Track 5 of the transcript/audio.** In the 2017 Com-Res survey for the BBC, a significant number of those who described themselves as Christian said that they didn't believe in the Resurrection. In your view, is belief in the Resurrection fundamental to being a Christian?

7. **Read Luke 10.1-5.** Some people try to create opportunities to talk about their faith. Do you? If not, what holds you back? Do you know any 'natural evangelists'?

8. **Read Matthew 28.20; track 3 of the audio/transcript.** A key aspect of the Easter message is that the risen Christ is with us always – during dark times and joyful times. How does that relate to your own experience?

9. **Read Luke 5.18-20; track 5 of the audio/transcript.** Ruth Gee is sustained by the worshipping community: '[Faith] doesn't all depend on me. I'm a Christian in the company of others.' How important are church-going and Christian fellowship for your faith?

10. **Read Romans 12.1-2 & 2 Corinthians 5.17-18.** See Giles Fraser's words in the box on p. 1. One of Bishop John's main reasons for believing in the Resurrection is the transformation of the disciples. Do you know of any modern Christians whose lives have been turned around by the risen Christ? Has yours?

11. **On track 4 of the audio/transcript** our contributors discuss where they bump into the risen Christ. Have you ever 'bumped into' the risen Christ? Where?

12. **On track 5 of the audio/transcript** Paul Vallely says he thinks about faith as a 'process', a 'journey', even a 'roller-coaster'. Is that true for you? How do you think about faith?

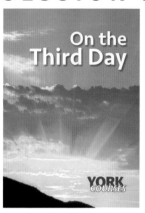

On the Third Day

YORK
COURSES

SO WHAT? The implications of the resurrection

It was the 1960s and the Anglican Bishop of Southwark Mervyn Stockwood, was in Moscow over the Easter season. He went to the hair salon of his hotel for a shave because his electric razor had broken. The hairdresser saw his episcopal cross and ring and asked him if he was a bishop. He agreed that he was. The hairdresser took his cross and kissed it and did the same with his ring. She then held the razor aloft with the bishop's beard still on it, and called out, 'Christ is risen!' whereupon the other customers joyfully responded, 'He is risen indeed. Alleluia!' Mervyn Stockwood thought to himself, 'Poor old Brezhnev [then Soviet President]: 60 years of atheism and still the Galilean conquers!'

Such is the effect of the resurrection. Its implications are extraordinary and the resurrection continues to ricochet around the world. But let's start with the basics. What does this event mean?

1. **Death is defeated.** Death has always been seen by humanity as an enemy. As the writer Julian Barnes put it: 'Death never lets you down, it remains on call seven days a week and is happy to work three consecutive night shifts. You would buy shares in it if they were available.' But the resurrection of Jesus assures us that even though death is still an enemy, it's now a defeated enemy. The tyrannical gates have been broken open; the people are pouring through, shouting their slogans of freedom.

Easter is the day death died and we have the assurance that heaven awaits (1 Corinthians 15.12). There is life after death, a life we hardly dared hope for, and the context is nothing less than a new heaven and a new earth, with Christ at the centre. It's hard to hold on to such a fantastic vision in a culture that desperately tries to avoid death, the great uncertainty, 'the dark wind blowing from the future' (Albert Camus). But there it is. In such a culture the resurrection is a blast of fresh air. Death is irrevocably defeated. (1 Corinthians 15.26.)

2. **Jesus is vindicated as the Messiah, the Son of God.** Who Jesus was had been disputed throughout his life. Was he the Messiah, the great military leader long awaited, or just a great teacher or perhaps a prophet. Nor did Jesus make it any easier. He refused to claim

> It is never too late to be what you might have been.
>
> *George Eliot, novelist*

> There was that essential belief that my soul lay in the hands of God and couldn't be taken by others.
>
> *Terry Waite, talking about his years in captivity*

> You never see further than your headlights, but you can make the whole trip that way.
>
> *Professor E L Doctorow, writer*

pray each day. I talk to
esus, I live with Jesus, I
valk with Jesus, I want
o be like Jesus, I want to
earn from Jesus. Jesus and
he are always together.
Archbishop Desmond Tutu

our life may be the only
ible someone reads. You
re the Fifth Gospel.
Mark Russell, Chief
Executive of the
Church Army

h Western Europe we have
ong been preoccupied
vith sin and death and
vith what sin and death
lid to Christ, instead of
eing preoccupied with
hrist, and with what
hrist did to sin and death.
The Very Revd
Michael Stancliffe

Most of the students
oreparing for Christian
ninistry] I now teach
ave had to defend their
lecision to believe in
iod against mockery and
ncredulity, so their faith
las a hard-won depth that
nay have been lacking in
orevious generations.
Jane Williams,
Tutor in Theology

the title of Messiah, still less the status of divinity, as Son of God, although he did many of the things that fitted that belief like a glove, such as forgive sins, rewrite bits of Jewish law, say he would be judge on the Last Day and so on. 'Are you the Son of God?' he was asked at his 'trial'. 'You say that I am,' he replied. They had to see it for themselves.

There were false messiahs in abundance in those days. Tom Wright names twelve in Jesus' time alone and is able to record their deaths. But no follower of those messiahs continued to believe in their so-called messiah after he'd been crucified - that was the end of it. Not so with Jesus. His followers were turned inside out and upside down, and then exploded into the world with a message of resurrection. There was no more hesitation – Jesus was the Messiah, the Son of God.

3. The Cross is a victory, not a defeat. It looked pretty grim that Good Friday night. Jesus was a bloody corpse in a grave; the disciples were hiding out wherever they could; the women were shell-shocked, knowing only that they must buy spices for the body. It was all disastrous: the Galilean dream was shattered. But on the third day all that was reversed. Very soon those believers came to see that the cross had not been a brutal defeat after all, but a glorious victory.

Traditionally we've said it was a victory over sin and death (1 Corinthians 15.55,56). It's easy to see that it was a victory over death because Jesus was alive, but what about a victory over sin? Sin was present in all sorts of miserable ways on the cross; so much evil was being unleashed on Jesus – the hatred, cruelty and violence of the perpetrators, the lust for power, the corruption of leaders, the selfishness, arrogance and vanity of humankind, the shoddiness of religion. It was all flying at Jesus. And he took it without flinching, absorbed it without reproach. He returned love for hate, forgiveness for cruelty. He took it into himself, soaked it up, and so in a sense he disarmed the powers of darkness at their strongest point. Love conquered.

When one of our children was very small, she would sometimes get into such a rage that all you could do as a parent was open your arms and hold the furious little body - taking the punishment, absorbing the

A great deal more failure is the result of an excess of caution than of bold experimentation with new ideas. The frontiers of the kingdom of God were never advanced by men and women of caution.

Oswald Saunders, missionary

Our Lord has written the promise of resurrection, not in books, but in every leaf in springtime.

Martin Luther, reformer

It's not that I'm afraid to die. I just don't want to be there when it happens.

Woody Allen

Where is God? God isn't just in the church building, God is out in the fields with the horses, with the storytellers around the camp fire. God is within us, in our culture, in our language, in the celebration of who we are.

Tracey-Jane Anderson (Reader)

anger - until she flopped, all passion spent. Victory, b at a high cost. So also was the cross a victory, and it was the resurrection that revealed it.

When Archbishop Janani Luwum was murdered by President Idi Amin in Uganda the authorities refused to release the body, and at the funeral the people were lost. Then the new Archbishop began to read the resurrection story in Luke, particularly the part where the angels say to the women, 'Why do you look for the living among the dead?' (Luke 24.5-6.) Gradually people began to realise the significance of this passage and a song of praise rose up all around the hillside, 'Glory, glory, alleluia!' they sang. The resurrection demonstrated to them, joyfully, that the cross was the place of victory.

4. **We've seen the beginning of the End.** Because of the resurrection we've glimpsed the goal of history, journey's end, the new creation. In the middle of history the End has begun. In the risen body of Jesus we see the tip of the iceberg of a new world, one which isn't a pale, pink-mist imitation of our current one, but a full-blooded re-creation of God's purpose the Kingdom of God. In the cross and resurrection Jesus took creation with him through the decay of death and out the other side, beyond the reach of death. Until now, creation has been groaning in labo pains for its new birth (Romans 8.22). Now we've see the point of it all; there's a Kingdom coming and we' seen the beginning of the End – so let's keep buildin

5. **Christ is alive.** It's obvious, but it needs saying. Someone I know very well, read and thought hard about the truth of the resurrection - and finally came away convinced. And then, she reasoned, if Christ ha been raised from the dead, he is still alive. And if he i alive, he could be known. And if he could be known, he could be her friend! The lovely truth is that we are never alone. Of course that doesn't mean that nothir bad will happen to us. In a world of cause and effect, of action and interaction, of chance and necessity, ba things may well happen to us. It's the way the world is, and has to be, if we're to be genuinely free. *But whatever happens, we will never be alone in it.* In the simple words of the old James Taylor song, 'You've g a friend.'

There are, of course, many other implications of the resurrection, some of which we'll return to in a later session, implications of both a more personal and a more overtly social and political nature. But we need to start with the basics, which are both personal and universal – the defeat of death; the vindication of Jesus; the victory of the cross; the beginning of the End, the true purpose of life; the presence of the living Christ, with us always.

Perhaps above all, we now know that life makes sense. We know that life isn't 'a tale told by an idiot, full of sound and fury, signifying nothing'. We are, by nature, makers of meaning, and instinctively resist the idea that life is nonsense. The resurrection confirms this instinct. It says we live in a fabulous framework, that of eternity, and we have a Kingdom to create here and now, one of love, justice and joy. What could give life more meaning and purpose?

Perhaps we should all take a leaf out of Mr Wrigley's book. Instead of the usual greeting we give each other: 'Hi, how you doing?' 'I'm good, how are you?' Christians should greet each other: 'Christ is risen, John!' 'He's risen indeed, Simon. Alleluia!'

he resurrection is not defeat needing the esurrection to reverse :, but a victory which he resurrection quickly ollows and seals.

Michael Ramsey, former Archbishop of Canterbury

hrist has forced open a loor that has been locked ince the death of the first nan. He has met, fought nd beaten the King of Death. Everything is lifferent because he has lone so.

C S Lewis

ife is a poor, bare thing vithout the sap of Christ's esurrection life flowing hrough it.

Terence Handley Macmath, writer

think that bitterness loesn't work – it damages ou more than it damages he other person.

Jenni Murray, broadcaster

The apostle Paul's greatest passage on the Resurrection is 1 Corinthians 15. He announces that the resurrection of Jesus revolutionises our outlook on the whole of human life – as well as on death. When we die we can look forward to being raised with Christ: *We shall all be changed; in a moment – in the twinkling of an eye* (v 51). In the meantime, even our humdrum daily work is given a new perspective. Paul was writing to slaves; for many this meant a life of tedious chores. So offer your daily work to the Lord, urges the apostle. This glorious chapter reaches up to heaven - with the death of death itself. It ends with a wonderful earthy anti-climax. Because Christ is risen: *Your labour in the Lord is not in vain* (v 58).

Canon John Young

QUESTIONS FOR GROUPS

BIBLE READING: 1 Corinthians 15.1-8

1. Bishop John gives five significant implications of the Resurrection. Is any one of these more important to your faith than the others? Can you say why?

2. **Read John 15.15-17.** On track 14 of the audio/transcript the participants differ in their responses to the idea of 'Jesus as a friend'. Which of these is closest to your experience and why? Does your faith work like this?

3. **On track 14** Tom Wright says 'friendships change and develop'. How has your relationship with God changed over the years?

4. **Read Luke 24.5 and Matthew 5.43-44.** Re-read the paragraph about Archbishop Janani Luwum on p. 8. Keep silence for 2-3 minutes and imagine that you are in the crowd at that funeral. Is there anything that you would like to share?

5. **Read Luke 23.34.** On track 12 Paul Vallely suggests that forgiving others helps us as well as them. Is this your experience? Are some things simply unforgiveable?

6. The poet Heinrich Heine allegedly said, 'Of course God will forgive me, that's his job.' Discuss!

7. **Read 1 John 3 and the words of E L Doctorow in the box on p. 6.** On track 13 Tom Wright suggests that the New Testament gives us true signposts into the future: 'but they don't give you more than a glimmer, a symbol of what it's actually going to be like when you get there.' Does this lack of clarity present a challenge for your faith? Or is it perhaps the essence of faith?

8. **Read 1 Corinthians 15.54-55** whic tells us that death has been defeate On track 10 Ruth Gee says: 'I a completely confident that I am love by God and so perhaps, in the en I will continue to exist only as o loved eternally by God. But that's n bad.' How confident are you that yc - and your loved ones - will live c after death? Does this include no believers?

9. **Read Romans 8.11.** On track 13 the audio/transcript the participar talk about how they imagine life aft death. Which viewpoint are you mc drawn to, and why?

10. Speaking about prayer, on track 14 the audio/transcript, Paul Vallely sa 'You don't get the answer in a form words, to a question in a form of worc When you get an answer in prayer i an insight or a resolution, and you fe "yes, now I know".' How does this rela to your experience? How does Gc answer your prayers - if he does?

11. **Read Isaiah 43.18-19 and Corinthians 15.52.** The Resurrectic tells us that everything will l transformed, including us. So hang c to your hat! Is this utter nonsense - the deepest wisdom?

12. **Read Romans 8.28 and George Elio words in the box on p. 6.** It's said th in (later) life we regret the things th we didn't do, rather than things th we did. Do you agree? How does beli that God is helping you to make th right choices affect this?

13. **Read Mark 14.36.** A young persc asks: 'If Jesus knew that God the Fath would raise him from death to glo why was he so reluctant to die?' Hc would you respond?

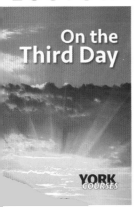

On the Third Day

YORK COURSES

'LET HIM EASTER IN US': Personal Discipleship in the light of the resurrection

How then shall we live? That's the pressing question of our time. And for Christians, that question morphs into how we should live in the light of the resurrection as the central motif of our faith. The answer, I believe, lies somewhere in the suggestive phrase of the Jesuit priest and poet Gerard Manley Hopkins, 'let him easter in us'. Easter as a verb – now that's intriguing!

1. We are an Easter people and alleluia is our song. The resurrection is God's love-promise to us, and the source of our joy. I once went on retreat as a young priest and remember listening to an elderly retreat conductor, full of white hair and wisdom, who looked at us and said, 'Never let the sorrows of this world hide from you the joy of Christ risen.' I've lived with that phrase for decades and found it to be profoundly reliable advice. There are dark periods; there are times when faith is dull, sometimes it's a struggle and occasionally it's very dark indeed. It's like exploring a mountainous terrain, full of high peaks and deep valleys; but at last we get the whole landscape, and the promise is that the final view is 'out of this world'.

So we mustn't 'over-claim' in our faith, making out that it's always a wonderful 'champagne and strawberries' experience. But the basic truth of our life as Christians is that we are an Easter people, given solid ground by the resurrection and on-going encouragement by the living Christ who 'easters' in us. The resurrection gives Christians a hunger for life. One of the key verses of my faith from the earliest days has been: 'I came that they may have life, and have it abundantly,' (John 10.10). The resurrection is the key to that abundance because, in it, the life of God simply exploded from the grave and flooded the world. 'You can't keep a good God down,' said a famous bishop, and we – Easter people – are the result.

2 We have new moral imperatives. Paul is clear in Colossians 3 that we have a new life in Christ that has important implications for how we behave. 'So if you have been raised with Christ, seek the things that are above.' (v 1). We have to put to death a whole list of destructive actions and attitudes (vv 5-9) and instead 'clothe' ourselves with compassion, kindness, humility, meekness, and patience. We are to bear with one another's foibles and forgive each other because –

Three things in human life are important: the first is to be kind; the second is to be kind; and the third is to be kind.

Henry James, novelist

Let him easter in us, be a dayspring to the dimness of us, be a crimson-cresseted east...'

Gerard Manley Hopkins, Jesuit priest-poet

A church that is not integrating environmental concern and action across its life has not fully embraced the ethical implications of discipleship having not fully understood the gospel of Jesus Christ.

Nigel Hopper, Baptist Minister

What the resurrection teaches us is not how to live, but how to live again, and again, and again!

John Shea, writer

Only when we see the bad news of 'man' in the context of the good news of God, can we help people cope with the anguish of living.

Augustine Hooey, retreat leader

The question of whether or not Jesus rose from the dead is the most important question in human life. For on our answer depends not only the question of whether or not Jesus was mistaken in thinking that he had a special role in the divine purpose but whether or not there is a divine purpose at all.

Bishop Richard Harries

never forget - we ourselves are forgiven. Above all we are to clothe ourselves with love and let the peace of Christ be our core motivator (vv 14,15).

The image of 'clothing' ourselves is a powerful one. In Romans 13.14 Paul encourages his readers to 'put on the Lord Jesus Christ'. I once saw a preacher do just that with a priest's surplice. He was dressed ordinarily and then, to illustrate the effectiveness of deliberately taking on the ways of Christ, he pulled the surplice over his head so that he was covered in that (strange!) fresh white clothing. I can see it still. We are to take on the character of Christ, be guided by his teaching and obedient to his call to live faithfully in our own age. We are not to be 'conformed to this world but transformed by the renewing of our minds' (Romans 12.2).

There are books and books on how all this works out in practice, but the key concept is that, in the light of the resurrection, we have a different starting point - a new basis for our moral imperatives. We march to a different drum. We unashamedly invoke the values we see in Christ and the vision of the Kingdom of God, that new creation of which we have now caught a tantalising glimpse.

3. **We have a transforming agenda.** The sheer physicality of the resurrection body of Jesus has significance. It means that the ordinary stuff of life is important; that matter matters. The resurrection body was no amorphous spirit, drifting around until called to higher things. There's a continuity from creation to incarnation to cross, resurrection and ascension that tells us that the material world is part of God's delight. Indeed, Gregory of Nazianzus tells us that, 'what is not assumed is not healed' i.e what is not taken up into God's life cannot be transformed by him. Every bit of creation is important to God.

So where does this take us? Surely to the conviction that Christians have a transforming agenda that includes everything - politics, business, financial systems, the law, economics, the arts, the environment, international relations, education, family life and so on. All of this is grist to the mill of building the Kingdom, or at least laying the foundations. We have a subversive social and political agenda to remake, transform and heal all human life under God. Christianity isn't 'pie in the sky when you die'. It's not 'in the sky' because we pray 'your Kingdom come *on earth*'. And it's not 'when you die' because it's already begun – millions of Christians are already at work on it.

In the dark days of apartheid in South Africa a political rally in Cape Town was once banned at the last moment, so Archbishop Desmond Tutu invited the crowds into the cathedral. The police and security forces trooped in with them, a sinister sight lining the walls of the cathedral. Desmond Tutu spoke. He said to the security forces: 'You may be powerful, indeed very powerful, but you are not God. And God cannot be mocked.' The diminutive preacher looked directly at them, gave them his winning smile, and said: 'You have already lost. So we are inviting you to come and join the winning side!' The place erupted. Archbishop Tutu was playing straight down the line of the Christian agenda of a healed creation.

4. **We offer hope to a world of confusion and low hope.** That story of Desmond Tutu reminds us that Christians are often amongst the few people who can truly offer hope. For us it's based on the 'impossibility' of resurrection. If we have a God who raises the dead then we can pitch our expectations higher than most! Indeed, almost uniquely, we have the full trajectory of past, present and future to bring to the table, while most post-moderns deal predominantly with the present and just take a punt at the future. As we seem to be spiralling into a future of multiple threats (global warming, religious terrorism, financial collapse, biological and cyber warfare etc.) we badly need 'a future and a hope' (Jeremiah 29.11-12). The resurrection gives us such a hope, and a sense of ultimate purpose. The world is not out of control; it rests in the purposes of God.

Hope is different from optimism of course. Optimism is passive; hope is active and intentional. Optimism doesn't need courage, whereas it takes a great deal of courage to hope when so much seems to be stacked against us. So the Bible isn't an optimistic book but it's full of hope. It's like Bishop Lesslie Newbigin's answer to the question about whether he was an optimist

To be a Christian means to be always young, in a sense far more profound than mere biological youthfulness. In the risen Christ, the Christian is always at the beginning of life.

Dennis Lennon, writer

It has long been my conviction that God is not hugely concerned as to whether we are religious or not. What matters to God, and matters supremely, is whether we are alive or not. If your religion brings you more fully to life, God will be in it; but if your religion inhibits your capacity for life, you may be sure God is against it, just as Jesus was.

John V. Taylor, former Bishop of Winchester

I feel very strongly that Christians should be involved in the public square. They should bring integrity, a focus on service, prayer and compassion. I'm very encouraged whenever Christians get involved to bring those qualities into Westminster. We want to be bringing them and bringing them in abundance.

Gary Streeter MP

or a pessimist, when he said: 'Neither. Jesus Christ is risen from the dead.' That counter-intuitive fact of the resurrection is what gives Christians the courage to offer hope to an anxious world.

5. **We can approach death confidently.** All right, death will never be our best friend, but in the light of the resurrection we can at least be sure of the welcome beyond. Indeed, when Cardinal Basil Hume learned that he only had two months to live he phoned a friend, the Abbot of Ampleforth, who burst out, "Congratulations! I wish I could come with you.' With somewhat more restraint, as he approached his martyrdom, Dietrich Bonhoeffer wrote: 'Death is the supreme festival on the road to freedom.' The point is that death is a busted flush for the Christian. It has its terrors, of course, but those are more to do with the process of dying than the fact of it.

The Easter message rings with confidence in a glorious life after death (or 'life after life after death', according to Tom Wright). We would be wise not to speculate on what this new life will be like – those who do so seem to offer a rather dull picture of life as we already know it, but with the bumps ironed out. Rather, this new life in God will surely be so far beyond anything we can imagine, that we should be genuinely excited at the prospect, but struck dumb at the description. It's sufficient that God will 'gather up all things in Christ, things in heaven and things on earth' (Ephesians 1.10).

And we are amongst the 'all things'.

> The royal doors are opening! The Great Liturgy is about to begin…'
> *Dying words of Prince Eugene.*

> What the resurrection of Jesus reveals is that there's a deep moral structure to the universe … anchored at its centre by ultimate love and power… you live life its way or it simply won't come out right.
> *Ronald Rolheiser, priest*

> This life is not all there is. We have been given the unconquerable hope of the resurrection; and much is required of those to whom much is given.
> *Revd Canon Angela Tilby*

> I told you I was ill.
> *Comedian Spike Milligan's epitaph*

Dame Cicely Saunders famously founded the modern (now worldwide) Hospice movement. It was a long, hard road and she said that without the teaching of Jesus to inspire her, and the Spirit of Christ in her heart to encourage her, she couldn't have pressed on to make her dream become reality. She needed the guidance of the risen Christ – and the inner strength that his resurrection brings.

Canon John Young

QUESTIONS FOR GROUPS

BLE READING: Colossians 3.1-4 & 12-17

- What would you like the epitaph on your gravestone to say?

- **Read Matthew 11.28-30.** Re-read point 1 on page 11. Group members are invited to outline a 'dark time' in their own lives. During that time, did 'the joy of Christ risen' help to overcome 'the sorrows of this world' for you?

- **Read John 10.10** - Bishop John's own 'key verse'. Do you have a key verse that sustains you?

- **Read Colossians 3.12.** It's all very well saying 'clothe yourself with compassion, kindness, humility ...' but how do you do that? Is it just a matter of trying harder and harder? Our participants discuss this on track 18 of the audio/transcript.

- **Re-read point 3 on p. 12 and the box on p. 14 about Dame Cicely Saunders.** Bishop John is keen to point out that the Resurrection has implications for all of life, not just the 'religious bit'. What do you think are the most important points where the Church and individual Christians should be at work in society today?

- **Re-read point 4 on p. 13; track 16 of the transcript/audio.** 'The world is not out of control; it rests in the purposes of God.' Yet our world seems to lurch from disaster to disaster. Can you square that circle?

7. **Read 2 Timothy 1.10.** Do you wish for/ hope for/expect immortality? In heaven - or perhaps on earth in some way? Do you think having grandchildren makes a difference?

8. **Read Mark 10.30.** Tom Wright says on track 16 that we should not expect the Risen Christ, 'to keep us in cotton wool'. What does he mean? Do you ever hope for or expect 'cotton wool'?

9. **On track 18 of the transcript/audio** Ruth Gee says, 'We have to bear with one another's foibles and forgive each other but that's not just a matter of forgetting, of overlooking, it's also a matter sometimes of challenging'. How might the message of Easter transform our relationships with one another? Does it?

10. **Revelation 21.4.** Ruth Gee talks on track 19 about death and dying. Is your Christian faith a comfort to you when contemplating death and dying?

11. **Read Genesis 1.31.** In her Closing Reflection Bishop Libby says, 'the Resurrection involves the whole of creation'. In the light of climate change, as an individual and as a church, how seriously do you take your own responsibilities towards God's Creation?

12. **Read Mark 8.34 and John 10.10.** On p. 11 Bishop John writes, 'we mustn't over-claim our faith, making out that it's always a wonderful champagne-and-strawberries experience'. But why isn't it? Our participants discuss this on track 17.

SESSION 4

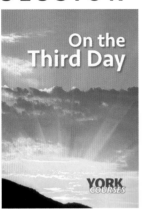

On the Third Day

YORK COURSES

CELEBRATING AND PRAYING EASTER

I saw a lot of working-class men and women – myself included – living a deeper, more thoughtful life than would have been possible without the Church. These were not educated people; Bible study worked their brains. They met after work in noisy discussion. The sense of belonging to something big, something important, lent unity and meaning…

Jeanette Winterson, writer

We spend a very long time getting ready for Christmas. It starts in early September as the first catalogues drop through the letterbox and people start telling you how many shopping days there are until Christmas. The Church tries to hold back the tide of commercialism at least until Advent, but eventually we have to enter the 'carol-service-and-nativity-play' season with a will and a sigh. Shepherds, angels and kings are all over the place. Little donkeys carry Mary. Stars twinkle over the stable if the electrician has done his job. And, in the middle of it all, 'the heavenly babe you there shall find' is trying his best to survive the fuss.

Then the day itself is one of hyper-indulgence that continues as long as the turkey or the budget holds out. The rituals, the lunch, the television schedules, the family gatherings … we know how to do Christmas.

But Easter? There's a slow and serious build-up called Lent, that society doesn't particularly notice. And there's a sombre seven days called Holy Week, that society would be embarrassed about - if it understood what it was for - followed by a family weekend of chocolate, daffodils and bunny rabbits. And then it's all over. Summer holidays come next.

How can it be that the greatest event in the history of the world makes so little impression? Even Christians seem to find it hard to hold on to the magnitude of the event, the sheer beauty and joy of it. Our liturgies do their best, the Easter candle is still lit, but the glory dies away and normal service is resumed with disappointing haste.

How can we celebrate and extend this King-and-Queen of festivals so that it resonates more deeply in us and penetrates more effectively into our Christian sensibilities?

Celebrating the day

I won't dwell on Easter worship. We usually do that well. There's joy, glorious music, extravagant flowers, an Easter garden, smiley greetings - and sun streaming through the windows if nature is doing its bit. Maybe there's a treasure hunt for chocolate eggs in the churchyard or egg-rolling down a hillside. We catch at least the edges of the Easter ecstasy.

We pray constantly to an
'Almighty God'. But do we
pray enough to a gentle
God who came to us as a
human being, born naked
and dying naked?
Alan Bartlett, priest

~

Pray for me as I will for
thee, that we may merrily
meet in heaven.
*Sir Thomas More (awaiting
his execution)*

~

The prayer of my friends
and the spiritual power
which seemed to pour
through them, was like
a light, defending me on
every side.
*Eglantyne Jebb, founder of
Save the Children*

~

The world we build
tomorrow is born in the
prayers we say today.
*Jonathan Sacks, former
Chief Rabbi*

~

Prayer is taking the chalice
to the fountain to be filled.
St Augustine

~

We ask for silver and he
gives us gold.
Martin Luther, Reformer

Some churches are starting to think of Stations of the Resurrection as well as Stations of the Cross. Different places in the church easily relate to different parts of the resurrection story: the altar as the tomb, the Easter garden for the first meetings, a doorway for the Upper Room (Mark 14.15), the central aisle for the road to Emmaus (Luke 24), the font for the Lake (John 21), the pulpit for the proclamation of the message (1 Corinthians 15), back to the altar for the weekly act of remembrance in Communion.

That's in church, but what about at home? Just as we have Christmas lunch, could we not have Easter lunch: traditional lamb - or fish as a reminder of the resurrection meals in Luke 24 and John 21? Grace can take the form of a reading from one of the resurrection accounts. There can be an empty place set for the risen Christ.

The home can be decorated in the Easter equivalent of Christmas decorations. Yellow and white daffodils are obvious but we could have yellow and white balloons as well, and streamers or ribbons flowing down in the hallway and living room, symbolising the new life flowing out of the empty tomb. And presents – why should Christmas have all the good bits? The gift of the risen Christ to the world is the greatest of all presents, so we could echo that generosity, but with greater simplicity than at Christmas, more symbolic of beauty, grace and simplicity – those hallmarks of the resurrection. Flowers, music, simple foods, pottery or other beautiful objects, life-affirming books, these are the kind of gifts that might speak of a graceful God.

Praying Easter

One of the main ways in which we can embed the meaning of the resurrection in our on-going post-Easter lives is through the way we pray. Here are a number of ideas to get the creative juices flowing.

We could start all our occasions of prayer, whether public or private, with the exchange 'Alleluia, Christ is risen! He is risen indeed, alleluia!' That sets the tone; it reminds and encourages us that Christ is truly alive for us now, and not just on one morning in a distant garden a long time ago.

Do small things with great love.

Mother Teresa

Good Friday is about suffering and sacrifice. Easter Day shouts joy and faith from the pinnacles of our places of worship.

Bel Mooney, broadcaster

The great gift of Easter is hope - Christian hope which makes us have that confidence in God, in his ultimate triumph, and in his goodness and love, which nothing can shake.

Cardinal Basil Hume

Prayer isn't a matter of asking for things and being accepted or rejected, it is a matter of adding one's energy – insignificant in itself – to the vastly greater energy that is God's love.

Peter Leigh, missionary

It is our choices that show what we really are, far more than our abilities

Dumbledore tells Harry Potter (JK Rowling)

I like the idea of starting our prayers with 'Risen Lord …' instead of 'Gracious God …', 'Heavenly Father …' or whatever else we commonly use.

What about 'practising the presence of the risen Christ' as a variation on 'practising the presence of God'? Brother Lawrence was the 17th century French monk who found God as much in his monastery kitchen as in chapel, and encouraged others simply to remember, nod or smile in the direction of God during everyday activities. I remember as a young Christian walking back to my digs at university and finding great pleasure in simply remembering the presence of the living Christ with me. Sometimes we 'chatted', sometimes we just travelled together, but this was something deep and true, not just going through the motions of religious practice.

This idea can be extended, so that we greet the people we encounter during the day *as Christ*, alive and before us at that moment. This is the Benedictine discipline of hospitality, beautifully expressed in the Rule as 'let all guests who arrive be received as Christ'. It makes all our conversations much more meaningful, even precious, although it can be exhausting too!

*

Another way of praying at the start of the day is by using the phrase of the angelic messenger in Matthew 28.5-7 who said, 'He has been raised, and he is going ahead of you to Galilee; you will see him there.' As we look ahead in the morning at the day's events we can repeat, 'He is going ahead of me into … [whatever the day's events are] … I will see him there.' That's theologically true anyway; God is always there ahead of us, we don't need to encourage him to turn up. But it can also give us confidence and hope, particularly if we're facing some tricky moments in the day ahead.

I love the prayer known as *St Patrick's Breastplate*, because it seems to me to be full of an Easter confidence that Christ is always present:

Christ be with me, Christ within me.
Christ behind me, Christ before me.
Christ beside me, Christ to win me.
Christ to comfort and restore me.

Christ beneath me, Christ above me.
Christ in quiet, Christ in danger.
Christ in hearts of all who love me,
Christ in mouth of friend and stranger.

Slave trade abolitionist William Wilberforce wrote to his sister one Easter: 'The day has been delightful. I was out before six … I think my own devotions become more fervent when offered in this way amidst the general chorus with which all nature seems to be swelling the song of praise and thanksgiving.'

It is love that believes the resurrection.

Ludwig Wittgenstein, philosopher

The sun is up early and ready to shine in – if you open the curtains.

St John of the Cross

In India, if a man dies the widow flings herself on to the funeral pyre. In this country the woman just says: '72 baps, Connie, you slice, I'll spread.'

Victoria Wood, comedian

He is the calm reassurance that the risen Christ is present in every dimension of our lives. We're surrounded and protected by the same Lord who met Mary Magdalene in the garden, the disciples in the Upper Room, Peter on the seashore and '500 at one time' somewhere else.

Light and dark

There's just one last thing. Resurrection constantly seems to speak of glory, victory, and a positive vibrant faith. And yet, for all of us at some stage in our journey, there's a darker experience as the vitality and freshness of faith seems to leak away. At those times it may be good to remember that the resurrection itself happened in darkness, in a cave, in complete silence, with the smell of damp earth and cold stone. New life starts in the dark, and sometimes the darkness lasts for a long time. Seeds in the ground may have a long wait before they germinate. Perhaps we need to allow for a 'lunar spirituality' as well as a 'solar spirituality'. After all, God gave us twelve hours of darkness as well as twelve hours of light, and the darkness wasn't a mistake. There are, said Isaiah, 'treasures of darkness' (Isaiah 45.3) for us to discover.

So the narratives, images, symbols and themes of the resurrection are rich in prayerful possibilities. We meet at dawn, we light bonfires, we go down to the beach, we decorate crosses, we light candles, we sing ancient prayers, we drink champagne, we dramatise, sing and dance. In as many ways as we can, let us greet the risen Christ, and long for the joy of Easter to overflow into the rest of the year.

May it be so. May we be limited only by the boundaries of our imagination.

I have an uneasy relationship with death and suffering, with grief and lament. Perhaps it's because my faith tradition is more comfortable with the light of certainty than the darkness of mystery and questions… I fight against the urge to explain or pretend or ignore away the darkness. It's uncomfortable to lean into the pain, to seek God there. I do not obey my sadness. I default to attempts to control instead of the free fall of surrender.

Sarah Bessey, writer

QUESTIONS FOR GROUPS

BIBLE READING: Romans 8.31-39

1. In 1928, the British parliament passed the Easter Act, which fixed Easter Sunday as the first Sunday after the second Saturday in April. It has never been implemented. Would you prefer Easter to be on the same Sunday every year?

2. **Read Philippians 4.4.** What are the best things you've experienced in church on Easter Day? Can you recall a particularly memorable Easter service (inside or outside a church building)?

3. What, if anything, do you do at home to celebrate Easter? Are there ideas on p. 17 that you like and might try?

4. Do you agree with Bishop John that to get the full experience of Easter we should lengthen it (into a season) and strengthen it? Our participants discuss 'rescuing Easter' on track 26 of the audio/transcript. What do you think?

5. Do any of the quotations on prayer in the box on p. 17 resonate with you particularly?

6. **Read Matthew 28.20.** Do you 'practise the presence of God' during the day – even if you don't call it that?

7. **Re-read the first 3 paragraphs** of *Praying Easter* on pp. 17/18. How do you address God or Jesus in prayer? Paul Valley (track 22) finds it easier to pray to Jesus than to God the Father - because Jesus has 'intuitive understanding' of our situation. Does it work like that for you?

8. **Read 1 Peter 5.7.** Ruth Gee ha experienced deep comfort throug prayer - and also a challenge t action (track 22). Can group membe remember a time when the experienced either, or both, of these? so, please share with your group.

9. **Read Philippians 4.6-7.** A fello believer asks: 'Why should I pray? If it right for me, God will deliver it anywa Discuss!

10. **Read Mark 12.30-31.** On track 23 Pa Valley is down-to-earth about our bus lives - pointing out that if we try to he everyone in need we'd either be a sain or overwhelmed. Can you describe time when you've been torn betwee one or more demands and duties? Ho did you resolve your dilemma?

11. **On track 24** Ruth Gee says she can fin a holding cross helpful. Do you eve find physical objects such as a cross, rosary, a candle ... helpful? What way have you found of focusing on th Risen Christ?

12. Tom Wright reminds us (track 24) tha in the Ignatian tradition, 'they sugges taking specific stories from scriptur and consciously imagining the scen with yourself as a character on th edge'. Your group might like to try thi using the 'Doubting Thomas' stor (John 20.24-29) or any other passag that appeals.

13. **Read John 8.12.** Re-read *Light an dark* on p. 19. Do you recognise th darkness referred to in the text Have you experienced 'the treasure of darkness'? Can you share you experiences of this?

Just one session to go! Think ahead to what happens when this course finishes ... Meet again? Another course perhaps? Organise a coffee morning to enthuse others? Group members might wish to use the *York Courses* booklet *Daily Devotional Readings from Easter to Pentecost*. (See page opposite for details.)

WHAT NEXT FOR YOU – AND YOUR GROUP?

DAILY DEVOTIONAL READINGS is a 48-page booklet with a thoughtful reading for every day from Easter to Pentecost ('Whit Sunday').

Ideal for individual reflection, it makes a perfect Easter gift for friends. (Lasts longer than a card - and more nourishing than an Easter egg!)

Last year some churches gave a copy of this booklet as an Easter gift to each member of their congregation. Specially reduced prices for multipacks at www.yorkcourses.co.uk make this possible.

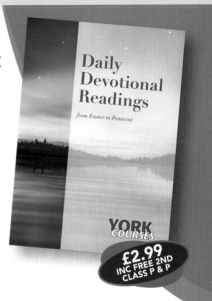

Daily Devotional Readings
from Easter to Pentecost

YORK COURSES

£2.99
INC FREE 2ND CLASS P & P

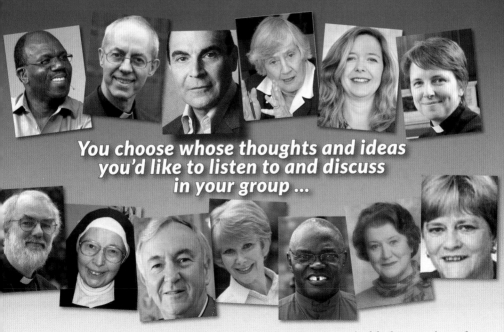

You choose whose thoughts and ideas you'd like to listen to and discuss in your group ...

We have some 25 ecumenical courses for discussion groups - suitable for any time of year (not just Advent and Lent) and we're adding to them every year.

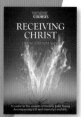

RECEIVING CHRIST

'To all who received him ... he gave power to become children of God.' (John 1.12.) This raises big questions. Aren't we all children of God anyway? What does it mean to have 'a relationship with God'? This course teases out from the NT various ways in which we receive Christ. St John's theology in his magisterial Gospel has practical implications for our day-to-day lives.

With Bishop Nick Baines, Margaret Sentamu, Revd Dr Ken Howcroft and Theodora Hawksley

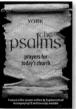

THE PSALMS

Course booklet written by Bishop Stephen Cottrell

These ancient poems have stood the test of time for they address many of the problems we still face: violence, injustice, anger – and bewilderment. This course reflects on the psalms in general (and five psalms in particular).

With Fr Timothy Radcliffe, Revd Preb Rose Hudson-Wilkin, Revd John Bell and Revd Dr Jane Leach

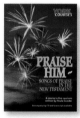

PRAISE HIM
songs of praise in the New Testament

Course booklet by Dr Paula Gooder

This course explores five different Songs of Praise from the New Testament – what they tell us about God and Jesus, but also reflecting on what they tell us about ourselves and our faith.

With Archbishop Justin Welby, Sr Wendy Beckett, David Suchet CBE and Moira Sleight.

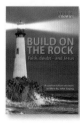

BUILD ON THE ROCK
Faith, doubt – and Jesus

Is it wrong – or normal and healthy – for a Christian to have doubts? Is there any evidence for a God who loves us? We hear from many witnesses. At the heart of a Christian answer stands Jesus himself. We reflect upon his teaching, death, resurrection and continuing significance.

With Bishop Richard Chartres, Dr Paula Gooder, Revd Joel Edwards and Revd David Gamble.

GLIMPSES OF GOD
Hope for today's world

Course booklet by Canon David Winter

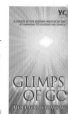

We live in turbulent times. This course draws on the Bible, showing where we can find strength and encouragement as we live through the 21st century.

With Rt Hon Shirley Williams, Bishop Stephen Cottrell, Revd Professor David Wilkinson and Revd Lucy Winkett.

HANDING ON THE TORCH
Sacred words for a secular world

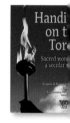

Worldwide Christianity continues to grow while in the West it struggles to grow and – perhaps – even to survive. What might this mean for individual Christians, churches and Western culture, in a world where alternative beliefs are increasingly on offer?

With Archbishop Sentamu, Clifford Longley, Rachel Lampard and Bishop Graham Cray.

RICH INHERITANCE
Jesus' legacy of love

Course booklet by Bp Stephen Cottrell

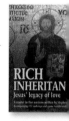

Jesus left no written instructions. By most worldly estimates his ministry was a failure. Yet his message of reconciliation with God lives on. With this good news his disciples changed the world. What else did Jesus leave behind – what is his 'legacy of love'?

With Archbishop Vincent Nichols, Paula Gooder, Jim Wallis and Inderjit Bhogal.

WHEN I SURVEY...
Christ's cross and ours

Course booklet by Revd Dr John Pridmore

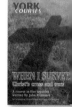

The death of Christ is a dominant and dramatic theme in the New Testament. The death of Jesus is not the end of a track – it's the gateway into life.

With General Sir Richard Dannatt, John Bell, Christina Baxter and Colin Morris.

"the York Course sets the standard for Lent courses ... it always opens up discussion." *Church Times* reviewer

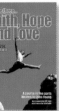

These three...
FAITH, HOPE & LOVE

Based on the three great qualities celebrated in 1 Corinthians 13. This famous passage begins and ends in majestic prose. Yet it is practical and demanding. St Paul's thirteen verses take us to the heart of what it means to be a Christian.

With Bp Tom Wright, Anne Atkins, the Abbot of Worth and Professor Frances Young.

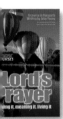

THE LORD'S PRAYER
praying it, meaning it, living it

In the Lord's Prayer Jesus gives us a pattern for living as his disciples. It also raises vital questions for our world in which 'daily bread' is uncertain for billions and a refusal to 'forgive those who trespass against us' escalates violence.

With Canon Margaret Sentamu, Bishop Kenneth Stevenson, Dr David Wilkinson and Dr Elaine Storkey.

CAN WE BUILD A BETTER WORLD?

We live in a divided world and with a burning question. As modern Christians can we – together with others of good will – build a better world? Important material for important issues.

With Archbishop John Sentamu, Wendy Craig, Leslie Griffiths and five Poor Clares from BBC TV's 'The Convent'.

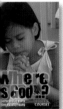

WHERE IS GOD...?

To find honest answers to these big questions we need to undertake some serious and open thinking. Where better to do this than with trusted friends in a study group around this course?

With Archbishop Rowan Williams, Patricia Routledge CBE, Joel Edwards and Dr Pauline Webb.

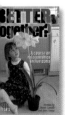

BETTER TOGETHER?

Course booklet by Revd David Gamble

All about relationships – in the church and within family and society. Better Together? looks at how the Christian perspective may differ from that of society at large.

With the Abbot of Ampleforth, John Bell, Nicky Gumbel and Jane Williams.

TOUGH TALK
Hard Sayings of Jesus

Looks at many of the hard sayings of Jesus in the Bible. His uncomfortable words need to be faced if we are to allow the full impact of the gospel on our lives.

With Bishop Tom Wright, Steve Chalke, Fr Gerard Hughes SJ and Professor Frances Young.

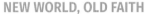

NEW WORLD, OLD FAITH

How does Christian faith continue to shed light on a range of issues in our changing world, including change itself? This course helps us make sense of our faith in God in today's world.

With Abp Rowan Williams, David Coffey, Joel Edwards, John Polkinghorne and Dr Pauline Webb.

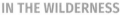

IN THE WILDERNESS

Like Jesus, we all have wilderness experiences. What are we to make of these challenges? In the Wilderness explores these issues for our world, for the church, and at a personal level.

With Cardinal Cormac Murphy-O'Connor, Archbishop David Hope, Revd Dr Rob Frost, Roy Jenkins and Dr Elaine Storkey.

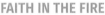

FAITH IN THE FIRE

When things are going well our faith may remain untroubled, but what if doubt or disaster strike? Those who struggle with faith will find they are not alone.

With Abp David Hope, Rabbi Lionel Blue, Steve Chalke, Revd Dr Leslie Griffiths, Ann Widdecombe MP and Lord GeorgeCarey.

JESUS REDISCOVERED

Re-discovering who Jesus was, what he taught, and what that means for his followers today. Some believers share what Jesus means to them.

With Paul Boateng MP, Dr Lavinia Byrne, Joel Edwards, Bishop Tom Wright and Archbishop David Hope.

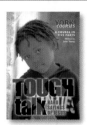

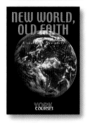

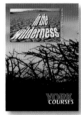

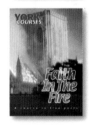

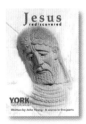

SESSION 5

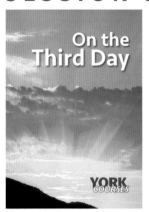

On the Third Day

YORK
COURSES

A RISEN CHURCH

I once celebrated Easter morning in the glorious setting of Canterbury Cathedral. The place was packed; the sun poured in through the elegant windows; the music was fabulous. My daughter smiled at me as I came down the aisle in procession, and I wept. Who could doubt that Christ was risen? Next Sunday I celebrated Communion under a solitary tree in the middle of the Sinai desert with a handful of pilgrims, three Bedouin tribesmen and four bored camels. But as we sang 'Thine be the glory, risen, conquering Son' it was the same Lord and the same joy. As another hymn puts it: 'One Church, one faith, one Lord.'

A risen Lord needs a risen Church, a Church that reflects the dynamic event that started it all off. The resurrection was like a huge explosion at the heart of history and we've been exploring the debris ever since - using it to build our all-too-human constructions of belief and practice in what we call 'the Church'. So the Church is built out of resurrection material. It needs to reflect its risen Lord.

As we all know, this is work in progress. We've done some disastrous things in the name of Christ. But what are we aiming at? What might a risen Church look like?

Joyful. The atheist philosopher Nietzsche wrote: 'I might believe in the Redeemer if his followers looked more redeemed.' Sadly we British often don't. We don't express joy like other cultures do by dancing, singing or laughing out loud; on a good day we might perhaps stretch to a slight twitch of the upper lip. And yet this faith we celebrate should give us a deep down smile in the presence of a Lord who lives forever with us and for us. I don't mean that Christians ought to grin inanely and share 'high fives' at the Peace; rather that we might cherish the risen Christ with serious joy from a deep place. I'd like us to be a Church that glows in the dark.

When the Russians went into Czechoslovakia in 1968 to put down the nationalist uprising they turned cathedrals into museums. A university lecturer took a job as a cleaner in one of the cathedrals so that the building would continue to be prayed in. For 20 years she prayed 'Be not afraid. Sing out for joy. Christ is risen – alleluia!' Joy stayed alive in that place. It's one of the chants they sing now at Taizé.

> To be a political leader - especially of a progressive, liberal party in 2017 - and to live as a committed Christian, to hold faithfully to the Bible's teaching, has felt impossible for me.
> *Tim Fallon (resigning as Liberal Democrat Leader, June 2017)*

> God does not coerce into joy, but there's always more on offer than we can take.
> *Professor David Ford*

> Be not afraid. Sing out for joy. Christ is risen. Alleluia!
> *Sung regularly at Taizé*

The apostles never regarded the Church as a kind of thing-in-itself. Their faith was in God, who had raised Jesus from the dead, and they knew the power of his resurrection to be at work in them and their fellow believers.

Michael Ramsey, former Archbishop of Canterbury

On the Day of Judgement you will be called to account for every good thing you did not enjoy.

The Talmud

Herod: 'I do not wish him to raise the dead. I forbid him to do that. This man must be found and told that I forbid him to raise the dead. Where is this man?'

Courtier: 'He is in every place, my Lord, but it is hard to find him.'

Oscar Wilde (in Salome)

Don't take care, take risks!

Canon Andrew White ('the Vicar of Baghdad')

Life-affirming. As we saw in Session 3, the physicality of the resurrection means that the ordinary stuff of life is important, that matter matters. The Church is too often seen as a negative, even repressive, organisation - instead of one intoxicated with the abundance of life we've been given by the risen Christ. Easter Christians will want to be involved in the whole warp and weft of our social fabric, affirming life and wanting to make the world better. In the Acts of the Apostles we see the beginnings of a Church where Christians got everywhere and lived differently – and thereby changed society from the inside out. That's been our life-affirming task ever since.

At the end of Matthew's gospel we see Jesus sending out his followers to *all* nations, with *all* authority, to teach *all* that he had told them. There was nothing small-minded, unambitious or narrow about this commission. Nor was the promise that went with it – that he would be with them *all* the time (Matthew 28.18-20). I love it when I see Christians getting involved in politics and social action, Christians taking their faith into boardrooms and offices, Christians working out their faith in relation to shopping, family time, hobbies, sex, the environment, the rest of life. I love it when I see Christians having FUN!

Flexible. Rowan Williams wrote of the Church that it is 'the community of those who have been immersed in Jesus' life, overwhelmed by it. Those who are baptised have disappeared under the surface of Christ's love and reappeared as different people.' If we are genuinely soaked in the risen life of Christ we can't re-emerge as stiffened versions of our secular selves. We must surely be developing the supple grace that comes from dancing with our divine partner. It's tragic when Christians are found defending all the wrong things and refusing the invitation to change. If Christians can't risk change, with all the guarantees of God's goodness and presence, then who can?!

When Mary Magdalene met the risen Christ in the garden she wanted to touch her beloved friend, but he gently forbade her. She had to get used to encountering him in a different way, one that was not less personal, simply one that was less limited in time and place, and allowed him to be available in *every* time and place. Can we not risk the same? Might not Christ meet us in a fresh, larger, more fulfilling way as we experiment with

In essentials, unity; in non-essentials, liberty; and in all things, charity.

Pope John 23

Churches are meant to be more than friendship groups or social clubs. … Church is based in the merciful sign of Christ, and love is found in the shared life of confession in which we find that ourselves and our neighbours are loved.

John Coutts, Tutor of Theology and Ethics

Jesus's teaching often offended the religious people of his day yet consistently attracted the marginalised and the irreligious. In the main, though, the church today has exactly the opposite effect. We often attract the religious, nice and upright people and exclude all those who don't fit. … Our message must be rooted in love, and we must be rooted in love. Sadly most people in society think the Church isn't loving. They think we are a bunch of judgemental so-and-sos.

Mark Russell, Chief Executive of the Church Army

new forms of church life? Indeed, the current dilemma of church structures creaking under multiple pressures looks like Jesus calling us on to new imaginings, less limiting and backward looking.

Why is it that an Easter people so often says yes to the theory but no to the practice? Why do we have such a sophisticated version of NIMBYism? I look for a Church that is, in Magdalen Smith's words, 'vibrant, changing, colourful, imaginative, loving, varied, merciful, challenging, hopeful and brave, even if it is also dark, fallen, bruised and fallible.'

Everyone a winner. I love the way that the risen Christ meets everyone after the resurrection precisely at his or her point of need. He met Mary at the point where she needed recognition; he gave her back her name, 'Mary' (John 20.11-18). He met the disciples at the point where their fear-fuelled hearts were making them live behind closed doors; three times he said 'Peace be with you' - and what he said in words he gave in reality (John 20.19, 26). He met Thomas at the point where his faith needed evidence because he had so much riding on it; so Jesus offered his damaged hands and wounded side (John 20.24-29). He met the disciples at the lakeside in Galilee at the point where they needed to restore fellowship with him; so he gave them a re-run of their special meal together (John 21.9-14). And Peter, of course. He needed to be reinstated in Jesus' confidence - and his own - after disowning Jesus three times; and Jesus met him with three questions that took Peter back to his first love (John 21.15-17).

*

Every person is unique and uniquely valuable in God's economy of grace. Every single person is made in God's image and likeness and therefore is irreplaceable. Everyone's a winner. The Church is at its best when everyone is welcome, no one is perfect, and nothing is impossible. One church was next door to a home where the residents had severe learning difficulties. Some of the residents came to the services but few people interacted with them. Until one Sunday one of the residents proceeded to take off all his clothes in the middle of the service. He was carefully taken out to the hall, but this dramatic event jolted the church into a proper recognition of the precious people who lived next door

e question to be asked
out every congregation
not: How big is it? How
st is it growing? How rich
it? It is: What difference
it making to that bit of
e world in which it is
aced?

Bishop Lesslie Newbigin

e East Harlem Sunday
hool was asked to
scribe the kind of
ople who came to
urch. 'Big people come
church,' said one.
hildren come to church,'
id another. 'Fat people
me to church,' said a
ird. 'Yes,' a small boy
ped up, surely delighting
s Maker's heart, 'and bad
ople come to church.'

*Revd Bruce Kenrick, social
activist*

each one made in God's image. The church developed a deeply compassionate and mutually fulfilling ministry from that moment on. A resurrection church includes everybody.

A Church that looks like Jesus. Christians are an Easter people with an ascended Lord in a Pentecost Church. In other words, they should look like Jesus. But how do you describe that? Perhaps the shortest and most accurate description is that it should be 'full of grace and truth' (John 1.14). But another description could be that it will inevitably be a *wounded Church,* just as Jesus after the resurrection remained a wounded figure, with the marks of crucifixion permanently in his hands and his side. We are the Church of the walking wounded, following a wounded Lord - but just as much as the individuals are wounded, so is the Body itself.

We can never find a perfect church because none of us is whole. The institution of the Church will be flawed, disappointing - even damaging, sometimes - because it is un-whole and still on the journey God has for it. Perhaps we should accept that we are part of the wounded Body of Christ, wounded by a thousand frailties, but still risen. And perhaps we might each hear afresh the question that the risen Christ put to Simon Peter: 'Do you love me?' And maybe we could say, 'Yes, Lord, you know that I love you,' and even, 'Yes, dear wounded Church, you know that I love you, too.'

And if sometimes we get more frustrated than we can manage, perhaps we could just say, 'Alleluia anyway!'

Because Christ is risen. He is risen indeed – alleluia!

iscipleship is a process of becoming. As people know Jesus better, through the Holy Spirit they
come more like him, more like the people they truly are. They are being transformed into his
eness. How effective the church would be at spreading the good news of this possibility if
eryone joining in was noticeably like Jesus!

Dr Katharyn Mumby

QUESTIONS FOR GROUPS

BIBLE READING: 1 Peter 2.9-12 & 23-25

1. Choose one of the margin boxes that you'd like to discuss.

2. **Read Hebrews 12.1. On track 32 of the audio/transcript** Tom Wright speaks about the immense value of Christian role models, while Paul Vallely reminds us of the importance of 'being normal in a kind way'. Do you have a particular Christian 'hero' from the past or the present – famous, or not? (It might even be a member of your own church.)

3. What do you think are the main changes the Church needs to make both nationally and locally in order to be a risen Church for our day?

4. **Read Tim Fallon's words in the box on p. 24.** You might also like to re-read Gary Streeter's words in the box on p. 13. Our audio contributors were asked about the key issues in society where the Christian voice needs to be heard more effectively (track 32). How would you answer that question?

5. **Read Matthew 5.16.** On track 28 Paul Vallely says, 'I think ordinary people look at the Church and think it's a weird place.' Do you agree? What do you think the world sees when it looks at your church?

6. **Read 1 Peter 2.9-10.** The Church of which we are a part is described as 'a chosen race, a royal priesthood, a holy nation, God's own people'. Does your local church/the worldwide Church live up to this?

7. **Read 1 Peter 2.11-17.** The N Testament describes Christians 'aliens and exiles'. Yet on track 32 l Vallely says, 'We have to come acros being part of the world like everyb else.' Is he right? What should ordinary, and what should be ex ordinary, about Christians?

8. **Read Matthew 5.14-15.** On p. 24 J Pritchard writes: 'cherish the risen Ch with serious joy from a deep place like us to be a Church that glows in dark.' Is your church life-giving and of joy – does it 'glow in the dark'?

9. A prayer often used at the end of a H Communion Service says: 'May we v share Christ's body live his risen What might a 'risen life' look like c Monday morning?

10. **On track 28** Paul Vallely descri a sign in America which said: '' church is full of hypocrites - but we squeeze one more in.' Discuss!

11. According to the poet Philip Larki church is 'A serious house on seri earth'. Does being serious allow ro for joy? How do you feel about laugh and clapping in church?

12. **On track 29** Tom Wright says he hopeful about the future of the Chu because of the risen Christ. Consi the current age profile in your chu and look ahead 20 years. What are doing right now to hand on the bat

13. Is there anything arising from course that you have not had chance to discuss, and would like raise now?

To end this course, you might like to say this prayer together:

May we who share Christ's body live his risen life;
we who drink his cup bring life to others;
we whom the Spirit lights give light to the world. Amen.

-SESSION COURSES

e audio material for these 4-session courses
atures Simon Stanley in relaxed conversation
th the author of each course - with contributions
m churchgoers of different denominations.

Ideal for Advent -

or any time

of year

PECTING CHRIST
tten by David Wilbourne

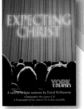

king at several moments in our faith and lives where a door opens
lets Christ in, catching the sense of expectancy which not only
es at the season of Advent, but throughout the year. In particular,
will be thinking about how Christ can surprise us and meet us in
distinct contexts: in family, in ourselves, in prayer and in the end.

JESUS: the voice that makes us turn
Written by David Wilbourne

Reflecting on Jesus' many voices: A Crying Voice, An Other Voice, A Dying
Voice, A Rising Voice. Four different voices that will make us turn in
our tracks and say to Christ, 'I want you!'

KING ROOM
tten by David Gamble

many of us life is full of things to do, people to
, responsibilities and chores. We can
etimes feel there's not enough time or space
the people and things that really matter –
uding God. New Testament stories help us
sider why and how we might make room for
at really does matter.

LIVING IN THE LIGHT
Written by Robert Warren

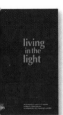

Practical steps in Christian spirituality as seen
through the eyes of four Biblical witnesses to
the coming of Christ. Exploring the 'reports' of
Luke, John, Mary and Paul engages with the
distinctive nature of Christian spirituality and
how we can give expression to it in our lives. This
course helps us to wonder, ponder and much
more.

WHAT ARE YOU WAITING FOR
tten by Lucy Winkett

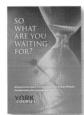

a cliché to say that we spend our lives waiting
life to start, but that's what many of us do until
realise that we've been living our lives all
ng! This course explores a spiritual life that
courages us to be active in our own time, but
ays rooted in God's time too.

Two 6-SESSION COURSES

GREAT EVENTS, DEEP MEANINGS

This course focuses on some of the most
significant days in the Christian year and
considers their implications for us as
individual believers and Christian
communities.

LIVE YOUR FAITH

This well-established 6-part
course is intended as an
introduction to living the Christian
life. It is designed for new
Christians, but also serves as a
refresher for more experienced
groups.

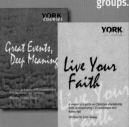

A FIVE-SESSION COURSE
for discussion groups and individuals –
suitable for Lent or any season

THE COURSE AUDIO brings the opinions and thoughts of these leading Christian thinkers into your discussion group. It's intended to be used in tandem with this course booklet.

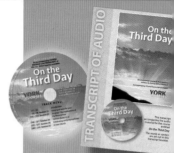

RT REVD TOM WRIGHT (Bishop of Durham 2003-10) is Research Professor of New Testament at St Andrews. He has written over 80 books and lectured widely around the world.

PROFESSOR PAUL VALLELY writes and lectures on ethics, religion and international development. A director of *The Tablet*, Paul writes for the *New York Times, the Guardian, the Sunday Times* and the *Church Times*.

REVD RUTH GEE is a former President of the Methodist Conference, and is Chair of the Darlington District, and also of the Methodist Council and Moderator of the Churches Together in England Forum.

THE COURSE TRANSCRIPT
booklet is a complete record of the words spoken on the audio material. Especially useful for group leaders as they prepare, it can also help group members feel more confident about joining in the discussion and catch up on missed sessions.

RT REVD LIBBY LANE became the Church of England's first woman bishop in 2015. Bishop Libby currently serves as Chair of the Diocesan Board of Education, as Chair of the Foxhill Retreat Centre and as Vice-Chair of The Children's Society.

OUR WARM THANKS to Julie Skelton c Appletree Design Solutions; to Katrina Lamb who transcribed the audio; to Jerry Ibbotson for recording and producing the audio material and to Linda Norman for proof-reading.

COPYRIGHT: © *York Courses:* August 201
The audio, the transcript and this booklet are covered by the laws of copyright and should not be copied. However, see **www.yorkcourses.co.u** for available discounts.

The image used for these course materials is copyright © jeka1984 – iStockphoto.com

The course booklet is written by **Bishop John Pritchard**, Chair of SPCK and author of 16 books on aspects of Christian belief and practice. He was the House of Lords' lead Bishop on education from 2010 to 2014.

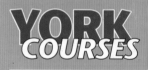

The course CD is produced by **Canon Simon Stanley,** co-founder of *York Courses* interviews the participants. He is a Canon Emeritus of York Minster and a former BBC producer/presenter.

York Courses · PO Box 343 · York YO19 5YB UK · Tel : 01904 466516
email: courses@yorkcourses.co.uk **www.yorkcourses.co.uk**

ISBN 978-1-909107-19-9

9 781909 107199